CHAKRAS FOR BEGINNERS

UNDERSTANDING THE 7 CHAKRAS, BALANCING
THE 7 CHAKRAS, AND STRENGTHEN YOUR AURA

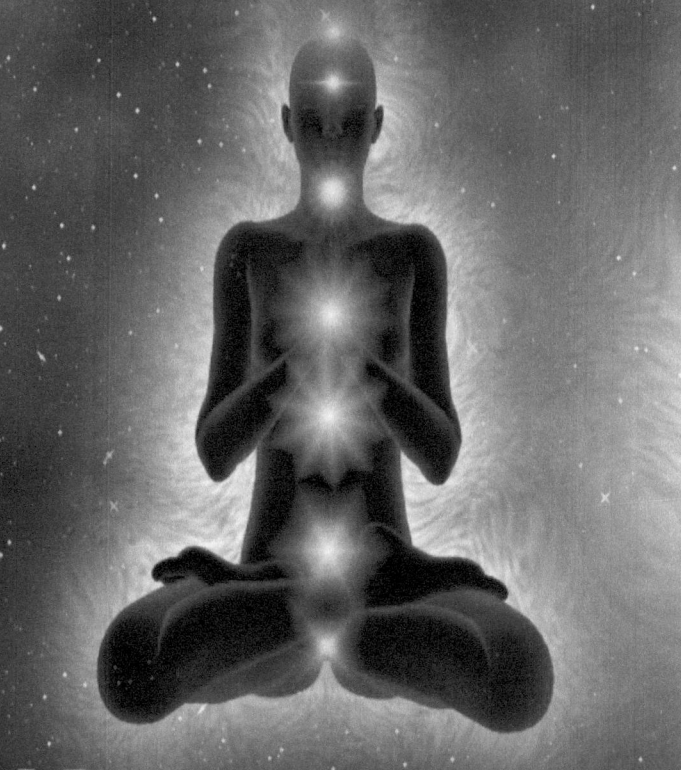

ABAHA SAAGAR

Table of Contents

Understanding The Chakras

Chakras are defined as spinning wheels of electric energy within you body. The wheels are responsible for functions that connect your body to your energy field and the broader cosmic energy field.

The seven major chakras include:

✓ The Crown Chakra – top of the head "Sahasarara"

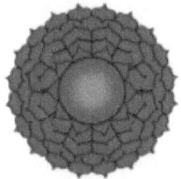

✓ The Third Eye Chakra – forehead "Ajna"

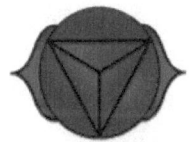

✓ The Throat Chakra – within the throat "Vishuddha"

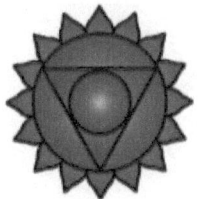

✓ The Heart Chakra – within the heart "Anahata"

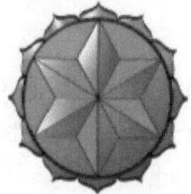

✓ The Solar Chakra – the solar plexus "Manipura"

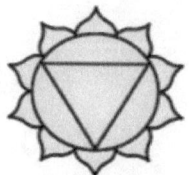

✓ The Sacral Chakra – the naval "Svadhisthana"

✓ The Root Chakra – Base of the spine "Muladhara"

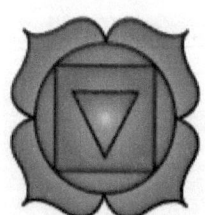

Each of the seven has their own different character and relate to one part of our life. This includes things associated with colors, the functioning of the body, elements, sounds and more. It is believed that the energy blockage that is found in the chakra is responsible to a number of different psychological and emotional disorders. It is a must that the individual have a good appreciation of the various chakras within the body. When they are not well-balanced, the individual suffers greatly.

Each of the different chakras plays a role in the way that we feel and the way that we respond to certain behaviors. It is essential just that each of the different chakras be well-balanced in order for the individual to thrive. But, that is where the problem starts. So many people in the world are not in tune with the chakras and are unable to energize themselves. They are unaware that they even exist, and when something goes wrong, like most people, they head to the physician in hopes that he can give them a remedy for their ails. While the doctor may be able to get something to you that provides temporary comfort, this is all that you will get. And, there are tons of different side affects that you also grind coming along with those doctor remedies. Furthermore you are not actually treating them when you see the doctor. Instead you are only covering them up for a period of time. This is not the way to enhance your life and it can actually cause Moe problems in the end. Rather than take these chances, understanding the chakras and how they can help you is a must.

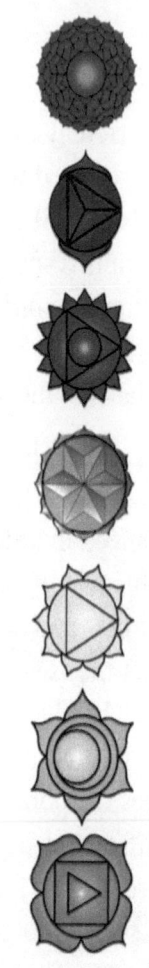

The chakras are linking mechanisms between the meridian system and the auric field inside your physical body. They also serve as a connection between the different auras and the cosmic energy field. The have a major impact on the flow of energy into your body.

The word "chakra" comes from old Sanskrit. The term means "wheel" or "round," and is used to reference particular energy focuses along your bodies centerline. The very first time that chakras were mention came from Hindu scriptures. The prophets mentioned the chakras as a pillar of energy that extends from the base of the spine to the top of the head.

Your body has one hundred in twenty minor chakras to go along with the seven major chakras.

7 Types of Chakras in Detail

There are a few different chakras within the body. In fact, there are seven of them. Now that you know a bit more about the Chakras, we will take a look each of the types of them and help you learn more so that changing your life and feeling better than you have ever before is something that can start as quickly as possible. We will also help you learn more about the roles that they play in the body, the affects they have when they are not in balance, and the different things that are associated with them.

"Sahasarara" The Crown Chakra – top of the head

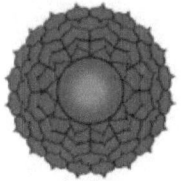

SYMBOL *"A thousand petaled lotus"*

The Sahasrara is called the thousands pedaled lotus. It is the element of thought and represents the colors white and violet. It is said to bring unity into an iniciusal and is located at the crown of the head. The mantra of the Sahasrara is at the crown of the head. This Chakra deals with the person's emotional feelings and integration of one's self. Physical dysfunctions of the Chakra include sensitivity to light and sound. The psychological issues with the Chakra include trust, apathy, ethics and materialism. When this chakra is well balanced the individual is able to maintain intelligence, is more open-minded and understanding and more easily able to adapt a variety of different information. Lotus is a related essential oil.

The crown chakra "Sahasarara" can cause a person to have difficulty thinking, a lack of concentration and a lack of empathy. Those who are not in tune with this chakra usually feel as if they are superior to other people and think that they are smarter than other people. Meditation is the most popular form of healing from this chakra. In addition to meditation, yoga and Tai chai are also beneficial.

With its location at the top of the head, the crown chakra connects to your central nervous system via the hypothalamus and the thalamus. The crown chakra governs the central nervous system, the pineal gland, the top of the head and the midline above your ears.

If this chakra is not balanced it could lead to chronic exhaustion, brain disorders, coordination problems, photosensitivity, mental sickness, epilepsy, ethics, and a lack of purpose.

"Ajna" The Third Eye Chakra – forehead between the eyes

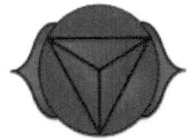

SYMBOL *"Descending triangle within a circle"*

The Ajna is the center of command. It is associated with the color indigo and is located between the eyebrows. Some people call it the third eye. This Chakra deals with the different feelings and thoughts of an individual. This includes their wisdom, intelligent level, detachment insight, understanding in, reasoning and more. This chakra, when not in balance, can cause a number of different physical attributes to occur. This includes eyestrain, difficulty learning, panic, seizures, spinal dysfunction, fear of truth, the inability to concentrate, headaches and nightmares. With a balanced Chakra it is possible to have a new reality and better concentration and focus. Mint and Jasmine help this Chakra.

The third eye, the Ajna Chakra, causes a number of different problems including those with the eyes, poor visualization, and a bad memory. It can cause a person to experience headaches on a regular basis, and even suffer with nightmares on a regular basis. Those who are deficient in this particular chakra are also prone to nightmares and hallucinating.

With its location between your eyes, the third eye chakra governs the neurological systems, the brain, pituitary gland, pineal glands, ears, nose and your eyes. The chakra has direct influence over your sense of trust, intuition and coordination. It has a direct influence over your sense of trust, intuition and coordination.

If this chakra is imbalanced you may experience issues with discipline, sleep disorders concepts of judgment and reality, emotional intelligence, confusion, blindness, stroke, seizures, brain tumors, arrogance, pride, learning disabilities and sleep disorders.

The third eye chakra enables you to put things into perspective and is key to learning and wisdom. This chakra is responsible for your intuitive intelligence and universal consciousness. Your third eye chakra helps you differentiate between reality and fantasy. When the flow of energy is blocked through this chakra, you experience a sense of distrust and self-doubt. An open and clear chakra enables you to connect with your inner wisdom and guides you in the choices you make.

"Vishuddha" The Throat Chakra – within the throat

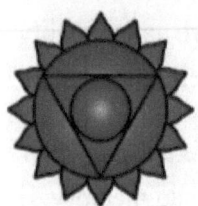

SYMBOL *"A circle within a descending triangle"*

The Vishuddha chakra is the purification chakra. It is related to the sense of hearing and is located on the nerve found in the throat near the pharynx. This chakra deals with learning abilities, responsibility for your own actions, faith, intuition and creativity. When this specific Chakra is not healed, there are many different physical complications that can arise. This includes swollen glands and gums, hearing problems, grinding of the teeth, ulcers in the mouth, swollen glands, tooth problems and more. When this chakra is balanced, as it should be, the individual is able to have positive emotions and expressions, good decision making skills, creativity and contentment. Eucalyptus and sage are the essential oils believed to benefit this particular chakra.

The throat chakra deficiency can cause fears, tension and neck stiffness. If you want to enhance this chakra it requires that you have a well balanced diet, participate in mediation on a regular basis, and of course perform yoga. Drinking water is also beneficial to those who want to energize this particular chakra. You can also do things such as shoulder openers, neck stretches and yoga poses like the Bridge Pose and the Camel pose to benefit yourself.

With its location near your throat, the Vishuddha chakra governs the mouth, gums, teeth, trachea, thyroid, vertebrae, neck, throat, esophagus, parathyroid and hypothalamus. It directly influences your sense of security, independence, self-expressions, loyalty, communication, planning and organization.

If this chakra is out of balance, the impact could result in the flu, fever, sore throat, swollen glands, thyroid imbalance, laryngitis, scoliosis, mouth ulcers, gum problems, vocal issues, tooth problems, faith, criticism, addictions, and decision-making.

The throat chakra is the center of your will power and communication. If you struggle to make choices or decisions it stems from this energy center. It also serves as the communication center with a divine power. Your faith is based in this energy center. Your ability to communicate the truth and voice your opinions is based on the throat chakra. With a clear throat chakra you are able to express your truth without any worries of what others may think or say. If the chakra is blocked, however, it will create anxiousness about how others react to your views and this leads to restraint.

"Anahata" The Heart Chakra – within the heart

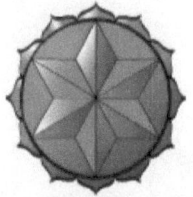

SYMBOL *"Intertwined descending and ascending triangles"*

This chakra relates to the sense of touch. It is located near the plexus of the heart and affects an individual's self-identity, their ability to provide wisdom and unconditional love, their ability to have patience and comparison. When this chakra is not balanced it affects the upper back and the shoulders, can cause asthma and heart conditions, lung diseases and the spine. There are also emotional issues that can surround an individual who is not balanced with this chakra, and this includes a lack of empathy, lack of compassion, anger and anxiety and even jealousy. When this chakra is balanced there is an empathic feeling, you are optimistic and free of resentment. Essential oils to help balance this chakra include lavender and jasmine.

This fourth chakra is the heart chakra. It separates the chakras from one another, and usually results in characteristics that affect an individual's way of spirit. Those who are defiance in this area are oftentimes shy and lack empathy. They do not forgive easily and oftentimes are anger and unable to form good connections with other people. There are a number of negative health effects that can result from this deficiency, including problems with, what else, the heart? Common problems include high blood pressure, heart disease and jealousy. To work on this chakra, yoga poses are recommended, including backbends and the Eagle Pose. While these things are beneficial, it is loving and the ability to do that that helps the most and offers the most powerful form of rehabilitation.

With its location at the center of your chest, the Anahata chakra governs the lungs, blood, circulatory system, thymus, diaphragm, heart, esophagus, shoulders, arms, legs and breast.

The heart chakra has a direct influence over compassion, forgiveness, passion, devotion, love for self, love for others, and your circulatory system. If this chakra is unbalanced, it can lead to issues like lung cancer, pneumonia, breast cancer, shoulder problems, confidence issues, envy, fear, hate, despair, confidence, passivity and jealousy.

The heart chakra is a storehouse of your energy system and the center of healing and love. This energy center is connected to your emotions and empowers you to give and love unconditionally. It also facilitates any emotional healing that is required and serves as a connection between your body and soul. You will feel connected to everyone in your life when this chakra is open and flowing.

"Manipura" The Solar Chakra – the solar plexus

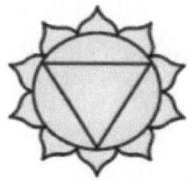

SYMBOL *"Descending triangle"*

The Manipura is the element of fire. It is related to the sense of color and sight. This chakra is found on the gastric or the solar plexus region of the umbilicus. This chakra affects the person's sense of well-being, their ability to understand and deal with emotional problems, stamina and the willpower and ego of an individual. There are a number of consequences of an unbalanced manipura charka. Those include diabetes, arthritis, stomach pain and stomach ulcers, low blood pressure, lack of self esteem, depression, inability to make decisions, hostility and poor decision making abilities. Some people also experience anger and bouts of rage. With a balanced chakra there is a great amount of energy, and the person is left with confidence and intelligence to make good decisions. This chakra, when well-balanced, allows for positive mental focus, good digestive health and better productivity throughout the day. Rosemary and lavender are among the essential oils that are said to enhance this chakra.

The Solar Plexus, or Manipura Chakra, causes a number of emotional problems such as low self-esteem, bad self-image and no energy. It can also cause anger, the need to be more powerful than another person and the need to be perfect and all ways. This can cause depression to develop as well as the person to need stimulants. Yoga is especially helpful for this third chakra, and participating in techniques such as the Half Boat Pose, Leg Lifts and the Boat Pose are all beneficial.

Located just above the navel, this chakra governs the upper abdomen, liver, pancreas, middle spine, gall bladder, adrenals, kidney, spleen, stomach, and the small intestine.

The chakra influences your self-confidence, growth, self-control, humor, self-power, ego power and digestion. If this chakra is imbalanced it may result in diabetes, constipation, digestive problems, ulcers, self-esteem issues, oversensitivity to criticism, self-image fears, nervousness and poor memory.

The Manipura chakra defines your self-esteem. Your mental awareness, ego, optimism, will power and confidence originate from your solar plexus chakra. The chakra is the energy center that rules your concentration power and your ability to comprehend things. Your natural instincts flow through this chakra.

"Svadhisthana" The Sacral Chakra – the naval

SYMBOL *"Up-turned crescent"*

This chakra is the element of water and deals with the individual's ability to taste. It is found between the genitals and the sacral plexus nerve. This chakra deals with emotions, creativity and pleasure of personal relationships. It governs the liver and gallbladder, the stomach and kidneys and the adrenal glands. When there is an imbalance in this chakra there is lower back pain, problems with digestion, menstrual cycle problems, hormonal imbalances, pelvic pain, feelings of being tired and problems with psychological concerns such as money, power and a lack of creativity. Those who have this chakra in balance are compassionate, satisfied with their sexual being, prosperous and humorous. The Amber and Orange Tourmaline gemstones are related to this chakra, as is the Sandalwood and Ylang-Ylang essential oils.

This chakra is responsible for your sensual and emotional well-being. When there is sacral defeincey there are many different problems that may manifest, which can include fertility issues, fears of change and even problems becoming intimate with other people. When there is a deficiency here there is oftentimes an exhibit of extreme emotional behavior. When you use the simple forms of yoga you can enhance the sacral chakra. You can do a variety of yoga poses to help here, and usually it is nothing more than a bit of gentle stretching that causes powerful sensations to be empowered to you. In addition to yoga, listening to music and aromatherapy are beneficial in this department.

With its location below your navel in your lower abdomen, the chakra governs the sexual organs, gonad gland, liver, stomach, gall bladder, kidney, upper intestine, adrenal glands, spleen and middle spine. It plays a major influence on joyfulness, enthusiasm, reproduction, and creativity.

If this chakra is imbalanced, anger issues may occur, apathy, hatred, menace, greed, guilt, control, power, immortality, pelvic pain, gynecological problems, urinary problems and libido issues.

The Swadhisthana is your creative center. It has influence in you finances, personal power, and your sexual center. This energy center connects you to your inner child, your feelings, and sensualities. It is tied to physical feelings of passion, love and sexuality. This chakra also facilitates the act of giving and receiving.

"Muladhara" The Root Chakra – Base of the spine

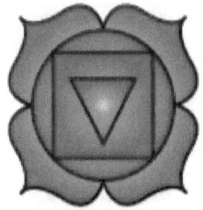

SYMBOL *"Square with a descending triangle"*

Muladhara is the element of the earth and affects the smell. It is found in between the genitals and the anus along the base of the spine. It deals with ambition, self-sufficiency, and stability, and governs the teeth, kidneys and sexual activity. Those with an imbalance in this chakra oftentimes suffer from poor sleeping habits, lower back pain, problems with waste elimination including constipation, being tired all of the time, anger, low self esteem, feeling alienated or possessive. When this chakra is balanced there is a feeling of independence, vitality and energy. Foods are digested much easier and you are overall much happier. The Ruby is a gemstone related to this chakra, and the cedar and clove are the related essential oils.

If you are deficient in the Muladhara, or root chakra, insecurities abound. This can be anything from money troubles to relationship problems that cause you to become insecure. When this happens you are probably feeling empty and lost inside, and anxiety creeps up on a continuous basis. There are even symptoms that can cause an individual to start hoarding and cause weight gain. If you want to help alleviate the problems that come with an unbalanced root chakra, one of the best things that you can do is a leg move during your yoga. Stretching the hamstring can once again balance the root chakra. There are many different standing yoga poses that can help you do this, and they also promote patience and calmness, so healing yourself mentally and physically is possible.

The root chakra governs the reproductive organs, the spinal cord, immune system, adrenal glands, rectum, and the legs and feet. It has a direct influence over your mental stability, sense of security, sensuality, and sexuality. If the chakra is not balanced, it could result in varicose veins, lower back pain, depression, immunity related disorders, rectal tumors, low self-esteem, and security issues.

Balancing the 7 Chakras

So how do you balance the seven? How can you balance something you cannot see? More importantly, do you even know if your chakras need opening or healing? Are they blocked right now? How do you unblock them?

These are very difficult questions with a very easy answer. To figure out if your chakras are blocked, all you need to do is look around yourself. How is your environment? How is your career? Are you satisfied with your health? How are your relationships? Are you satisfied with your quality of life? Take some time and meditate on your level of satisfaction with life.

The purpose of the seven energy wheels spinning from your spine towards your head is to channelize the energy wherever it is required. Each of the seven wheels links to a specific area in your body and also connects to specific situations in life.

The problem that can occur in life is that one or more of the chakras get blocked. You need to address the energy imbalance in your body, meaning that you will need to heal yourself through chakras and try and open up the blocked chakras.

Balancing Techniques

Yoga: Yoga works as an outside source to balancing your chakras by achieving physical and mental balance. It helps you concentrate through balancing your mind and enables you to achieve the perfect mind and body harmony. If you want to be your best then it is important that you are in tune with your chakra. All seven of them are just as important as the next, and it takes an imbalance of only one of them to cause you a world of troubles. Make sure that you are taking care of all seven of the chakras by participating in yoga and the other recommended steps to healing. It is a part of your well-being, you need the energy and there are good ways that you can get that.

Breathing Control: The easiest way to achieve calm is through breathing meditation. This will slow down your heart rate, which empowers your body and mind to slow down. If you want to achieve inner peace and tranquility, you must understand breathing meditation.

Meditation and mindfulness: Meditation has many benefits for both the mind and the body. It is a technique of relaxation that helps to condition the brain so that it actually functions better and communicates well from one area of the brain to another. Your mind becomes much more open for creativity, allowing you to use your creativeness and imagination easily.

This does not mean that only people who need creativity to create art, music, or writings should meditate; creativity can help you to think outside of the box, improve decision making skills by helping you to see more options, and even help you to see possible outcomes of decisions that you make.

It also helps in understanding ourselves, our feelings, and why we react in certain unwanted ways in order to reduce the stress that interferes with our lives. You learn to stop and quickly calm yourself when unwanted feelings arise, analyze your feelings or even put them on hold if necessary, and it improves your ability to think more logically.

Meditation cultivates a person in you that searches for peaceful understanding, avoiding confrontation. It helps you to communicate with others if you are normally direct or aggressive which helps keep yourself and those around you calm.

As a benefit of improved brain function, performance at work and academically improves as you learn to improve your memory, focus your attention better, and communicate thoughts and ideas. You become more confident in your abilities, which automatically strengthen them because there is less doubt in yourself.

One of the most important benefits of meditation is improved sleep. With less stress and the ability to let your thoughts from the day pass by instead of plague you for hours, it is much easier to fall asleep and allow your mind to work as your body rests. Restful sleep is very important to brain function, but many people do not realize that sleep can keep our bodies healthy and help deal with physical stress of illness. Another physical benefit is that reduced stress and restful sleep are tied to normal levels of cortisol. Cortisol is that nasty hormone that makes us gain fat, especially around the belly, and so one could say that it becomes easier to lose or maintain weight with meditation.

Energy Healing techniques: Reiki and acupuncture are the best energy healing techniques. They can help you open up your chakras once they sense blockage. They deploy specific tools that include crystals, gemstones, fine needles, pressure or touch and intention. Crystals are chosen based on the vibrations of these seven chakras. Pressure, touch or needles work through physically stimulating your meridians. Meridians are specific points that enable you to channel your energy towards the chakra. The most important tool here is intentions, which would imply concentrated emotions or thoughts.

Through the process of Reiki healing, spiritual energy is sent to your body: this in turn concentrates itself in areas that require it the most.

Color Therapy: Is there a certain color or colors that you prefer? Do some colors seem very soothing to you? Do some colors irritate you or make you feel off? This is not just a coincidence and it is based on the energy levels within your chakras. Every color possesses an explicit vibrational quality that can be utilized to balance a chakra in a manner that it resonates with the color. Do not forget, each chakra has its own color. You could use certain colors in your clothing or home décor. This can help support a blocked chakra.

Sound Therapy: Sound therapy works through the vibrations of energy within the ether. Have you ever noticed times when you prefer loud energetic music? Or times when you need some calming music for your mind. Listen to your mind. Your intuition will guide you to do what is right and needed. The problem many times is that we get stuck in bad habits. Classical music is a great source of music. In many studies it has shown a calming effect on ones minds. It also aids in chakra balancing.

Autosuggestion: Autosuggestion is repeated positive suggestion to ones self. You are what you think you are. When you repeatedly tell your subconscious mind something, eventually it will accept that suggestion as fact. That is why it is important to use positive suggestions. You mind is the most powerful object on earth. It willingly accepts positive and negative suggestions. We live in such a negative society that it is hard to overcome the bombardment of negative suggestions that we are exposed to everyday. Keep silent time for yourself and meditation time to focus on positive autosuggestion to aide in balancing your chakras.

Understanding Your Chakras

Chakra requires that each of the elements be opened and stable. Yoga as a method of healing uses different centers of energy from within the body. When the yoga is practiced, the individual is able to gain a better awareness of them; body, mind and soul, increasing the energy flow into the energy centers. As we have already discussed, there are a total of 7 of these chakras within the body. The chakras are responsible for awareness and are needed to keep our bodies balanced and our energy levels high. The key to being successful at chakra is to bring awareness to the mind by releasing various blockages that stand in the way. There are several different ways to increase the awareness of the chakra. For anyone who is looking to benefit with the form of the chakra, it is necessary that a deep understanding be met. You must be in touch with your inner being to target the various chakras in the body. When you are able to mentally connect yourself to this capacity, only great things can result.

Although all forms of yoga work to enhance an individual's overall well-being, using yoga to excite the chakra senses provides a far better understanding of yourself and the things that keep you energized. You are more in tune with your inner self and can develop a number of attributes when all of the chakras are well balanced and energized as they should be. And, yoga is a wonderful way to help yourself become more toned, mentally energized and feeling your best all the way around.

There are actually a number of different ways that you can enhance your chakras and feel your best. This includes through exercise, mediation, and of course yoga. This guide is designed to help you learn more about the benefits that can come with you when practicing yoga to enhance the chakras.

Origin of the Chakra

Chakras go back to the start of our being, the start of time. Tanzania, Africa, is the roots of the human race. There, Mount Meru exists, a large mountain that represents the journey of life. The top of the mountain is the Crown Chakra, the bottom is the root. It is here where the energy of the chakras was first developed. The mountain has been shown in Egyptian mythology, but it is from the Indian Tantra that the world today has developed much of their ways of doing things and the knowledge of the chakras and yoga to benefit them.

Chakras are something that we all have. However, it is not something that every person is in tune with. If you want to be a better person all the way around it is a must that you take all of the steps necessary to learn more about yoga and energizing the chakras within you. It is something that anyone who wants to change can do with only a bit of determination needed.

How to Energize your Chakras

Your chakras are stimulated every single day through various activities that you are participating in, even when you are not trying to do stimulate them. It is a natural occurrence that we are not really aware of most of the time.

Our thoughts and actions represent our sense and the way that we will energize those different centers. There are a number of different ways that you can charge the chakras in your body and ensure that they are well-balanced. The exact method of doing this comes through various yoga poses that you can perform. There are also various ways that you can energize the chakras, dependent upon which of them that you need to reinvigorate. Take a look.

Our thoughts are affected by chakras. If we allow positive energy to flow throughout our body then we are able to feel much better whereas the negative thoughts present negative energy and decrease the positive red flow of energy needed. If you are always thinking in a negative manner then you are taking every step toward lowering the energy of the chakra.

Our greatest energy source comes from the sun. All of the chakras are affected by the rays of the sun, as are all beings, including humans, plants, animals and water. If you are stuck in the house all day long, the chakras are not being energized, as they should. Getting out of the house as often as possible is one of the best ways to energize you and feel focused for the day. In addition there are methods of enhancing the natural sunlight in the home through the type of lighting that is being used. Ensure that you look at these lighting sources and use as many of them as you can throughout the home.

Did you know that the food that you eat also has an effect on the chakras? It gives us life, it gives us energy, and without ti the body is unable to thrive, as it should. You need to keep this form of the chakra in balance by eating foods that are a good source of chakra energy. Make sure that you eat foods that come from each of the seven colors of energy of the chakras to help yourself. This is the reason that people are so encouraged to eat a colorful variety of fruits and vegetables for the best health.

Aromatherapy is another awesome alternative therapy that will benefit you and each of the seven chakras. This is why there are essential oils designed to be used to enhance each of them. If you are interested in using aromatherapy to benefit yourself, then you want to ensure that you're using only therapeutic, quality oils designed for this intended purpose. There are a lot of fakes out there, so make sure that the choice is made carefully.

Listening to music is one excellent way to energize the chakras. There are few people out there who can say that music does not help them in many ways, including as a source of inspiration. It makes us feel good, feel bad, it helps us to relive a lot of different emotions, again, sometimes when we are even unaware of what is going on. There are many different sounds that can indicate energy to the chakras, such as eth sound of a drumbeat, while providing stimulation at the same time. If you are an individual who is ready to intertwine with their chakras, listening to music is a great way to get things started. It can relieve your soul in so many different ways that you might not have ever imagined possible.

Do you like to decorate? Are you someone that enjoys keeping his or her home up to date and designer? This can help you as you become more aware of yourself and your inner being. Yes, it is true, and if you are like most people you aren't even aware of the ways that the décor in your home can affect you. The décor in your home may be able to help energize the chakras. If you are using the right colors that enforce positivity, this may very well be an exciting, fun and easy method of exciting your senses. Try to decorate the home with the things that you like first and foremost, concentrating on colors that are all related to the seven chakras. You might want to use something such as a variety of artwork on the walls, different colored pillowcases or sheets on the bed, different carpet, etc.

The clothing that you wear also enhances and invigorates your mind. Many people are also unaware of this fact. When you feel good about yourself you are far more likely to take the time to care about your appearance and the way that you look to other people. You want to make sure that you are always wearing the things that you like, keeping in mind that it affects your energy level. When you want to feel great about yourself and have all of the energy of the day, wearing loud and vibrant colors is a great way to achieve this.

Enhance the Chakras with the right Foods

We have talked about the different ways that you can enhance the chakras, with a particular interest in yoga to enhance them. But, we have also talked about other methods of opening and empowering the chakras, including through the foods that you are consuming. It is so important that you are eating right if you want the best connection with each of the seven chakras. There are so many different nutrients that are found in the foods that we consume, when they are the right foods. Those foods enhance the brainpower that you have, and they also affect the way that you will feel. Let's examine some of the foods that you might want to consume to enhance your chakras. It is in your best interest to add as many of these foods to the diet as you can. There are a number of different ways that this can be done no matter what meal that you are trying to cover.

As we have already stated it is important that you are eating a colorful meal. The more colorful the plate, the healthier that it is, and the more advancement that you can do for your chakras. Each chakra is related to a color. Make sure that you are eating foods that contain all of these colors.

Important to remember when eating to enhance the chakras: no meat. If you are eating an animal you are promoting killing and other acts of violence. The entire purpose of chakra healing is to avoid negativity and bad karma. If you are eating animals you are certainly not using the power of the chakras. Rather than eating animals and meat, there are many healthy fruits and vegetables that you can consume to complete the diet. You will still get the needed protein in your body and also adhere fully to the power of the chakra and self-awareness of them.

Also keep in mind that it is oftentimes the root chakra that is the most essential in eating the right foods. There are so many problems that are caused at the root chakra, and without this well balanced meal, there are a number of effects that can result. When you change your diet to include foods that are beneficial to the chakra, this is not a problem that you will experience. Colorful foods are best to enhance the root chakra.

This includes red foods, with a particular interest in fruits and berries of this color. Root vegetables are also highly recommended, including yam. The chakra is a part of the earth. Foods that are symbolic with the earth and the soil are good foods that you want to include in the menu. Mushrooms are another excellent choice that can be enjoyed on a regular basis to enhance the senses of the chakra. The mushrooms are packed with protein and are from the soil, both of which you want.

Take a look at these favorite foods that you should enjoy to enhance the chakras. You're sure to find a variety of ways to introduce them into your diet, and you'll love them all!

Pomegranate: Pomegranate is another root chakra beneficial food that you can enjoy. This sweet fruit heightens all of the senses and tastes great!

Oranges: Another root chakra food beneficial to consume –oranges. What you might not know about oranges is that they can excite the chakras and all of your sexual desire and energy. So in addition to adding an enormous amount of vitamin C to your body, eating an orange will enhance your chakra and might very well cause a little bit of excitement in the bedroom.

Corn on the Cob: Corn on the cob is another yellow specialty that will enhance the chakras. Enjoy it as a nice side item with your favorite entrée.

Spinach: Spinach is a green, leafy vegetable with plenty of vitamins and minerals inside of it. Along with those qualities, spinach is also beneficial in enhancing the third chakra. With this enhancement you will learn better communication methods and will feel more positive each day.

Yellow Peppers: These peppers enhance the flavors of foods, but they do so much more, too. They can improve the functioning of your pancreas, which in turn also helps you with self-worth, your instincts, and more. Some people refer to this chakra as the third brain. Add yellow peppers to the menu as often as possible.

Kale: kale is another veggie to be included on the menu. This particular vegetable is beneficial to the heart chakra and helps the person feel love, empathy and similar emotions that we all need to feel. Kale can be combined with so many different meals, and provides an outstanding number of health benefits as well as a great way to improve the heart chakra energy and promote your well-being.

Blueberries: Rich in antioxidants, blueberries are the go-to snack when you want to enhance your third eye chakra. Regular blueberry consumption will give you a great boost of energy and help you mentally, too.

Beets: This red vegetable can be served raw or cooked, and offers a sweet taste that can satisfy your hunger. It is fiber-rich and high in antioxidants and enables energy to freely flow from the chakras.

Nuts: Nuts benefit the second chakra, and like most of the other foods that we have listed here are beneficial to the health in many other ways. They are a great snack that can be enjoyed at home or on the go, paced with protein that can fuel you for the day. Make sure that you have your favorite nuts (excluding peanuts) readily available at all times.

Water: Our body is made up of nearly 70% water, so, as you might suspect, you need it for proper bodily function. It is recommended that adults consume no less than eight glasses of H2O each day. This amount should be enough to suffice for what you lose in a single day. Water is lost from the body through numerous functions, including sweating and urination. Make sure that you replace that water and you will look better and you feel better too. There is nothing in this world that is healthier than water, so choose it any time that you need a great thirst quencher.

Your body needs a wide variety of raw foods to thrive properly. The 10 listed above are among the best choices that you have when you want to enhance the energy that is found within the chakras, but this is only a sampling of the things that you can enjoy to enhance your chakras. Along with taking all of the other measures of improving the energy that flows to the chakra, make sure that you are also carefully monitoring the foods that you are eating. When it is a well-balanced diet that you are eating on a regular basis, then you can be sure that you are getting what you need in your body. It can start with these foods. They are great for you to consume in more ways than one, certain to bring you into the energizing state that you desire to be in.

Avoid these Foods

There are a number of foods that should be avoided while living a chakra lifestyle. These foods can cause a number of blockages that can cause the individual to suffer. These foods are particularly harmful to the second chakra, the sacral chakra. One of the biggest is addiction to the foods, or rather, the substances found within them. Foods which are high in fat or salt should be avoided, as those with MSG. Caffeine is yet another of the avoided products if you want to enhance the sense of your chakra.

In addition to avoiding those foods listed above, make sure that you also eliminate smoking from your life, as well as the consumption of alcohol. As we are already aware, smoking is the number one cause of lung disease and many cancers, as well as responsible for many cases of heart disease. It ages you quickly, causes wrinkles and can also cause you to lose touch with the energy inside of you.

It is important that when you decide you want to become closer to your chakras that you are also making changes with the diet. The foods that are consumed have a major impact in your overall well-being, just as the chakras that we all have. When you are able to change your overall atmosphere the benefits are astounding.

Chakra: How to Get Started

While it would be nice if you could simply pop in an instructional video and learn how to do yoga this is not the way that you want to learn how to do things. Yes, it is an option and there are many people who do this rather than ever making a visit to a yoga studio. Not only are you causing yourself potential injury and damage by trying to take things into your own hands, you might also face the trouble of learning improper techniques, the last thing that you want to happen as you are trying to advance yourself and the life that you are liking. This is just the start of the many dangers that can come along with trying to learn yoga on your own.

Now, if you want to make the purchase of one of those DVDs that teach you yoga from the comfort of your home, this is an option that is available to you. But why would you want to cause potential damage to your life when you are trying to make great changes? Someone, somewhere, is looking to make money off of you through these DVDs. But, this is probably not the option that you want to choose, especially if you are new to the world of yoga. Not only do you need a certified yoga instructor to teach you how to do things so that you are not injuring yourself or hurting your body, it is also important that you are able to mentally connect with the chakra so that you can benefit, as you should be from doing yoga.

Tips for Success

Once you have made the decision to perform yoga and have chosen the studio that will help teach you, a few other things are in store for you to learn in order to fully benefit with your newfound teachings.

First, as we have mentioned countless times throughout this life, you need to be in tune with your body, as well as your mind. Some of the moves and positions of yoga are not for the light-hearted, as they stretch your body in ways that you might not have even realized possible for the body to move.

Have you purchased an outfit that is designed especially for participation in yoga? It is necessary that you are wearing clothing that is comfortable and easy on the body, and while it may not necessarily be the yoga outfit that you want to wear, they are a lot of fun to purchase.

While you are out shopping, choose a mat. The yoga mat is a very important piece of the puzzle of success. You want to be as comfortable as you possibly can as you are performing the various techniques of yoga, and it's with the mat and the comfortable yoga type clothing that you are wearing that will make a world of difference in things. Many different types of mats are available for yoga. They are made of various materials and constructed of various sizes. One of the mats can be purchased at an affordable price, and you want to make sure that you are choosing a good mat. Again, your entire experience with yoga is dependent upon a nice, comfortable mat and the clothing that you are wearing.

There is no way for you to know just what to do during the first few classes. So, it is okay to look and to listen, but make sure that you are trying. Take special note of the alignment of the instructor. This is one of the first things that must be done in order to conquer yoga. As you are looking at other people and observing what they are doing you will begin to pick up on things and better learn how to do yoga.

Finally, make sure that you take things slowly and never try to rush. Anything worth having taken time to achieve, and you should not expect those great changes to be made in a night or even in a week. The more that you are participating the easier that things will become, and before you know it, you will be a yoga pro! As long as you have patience and the eagerness and desire to success you can certainly do just that! No matter who you are, what type of background you come from or the ideal results that you want, they can be found!

Opening the Chakras

Just as you start participating in yoga, opening the chakras is a process that must be taken slowly. It is not something that you will fully grasp in a single night, nor is it something that should be expected. Understanding that there are chakras, and that you want to change your overall being, is the first step in identifying and connecting with the chakras that are within you.

To open the chakras that you have it is important that you discard all of the distrust that you may have, and that you are able to form a connection mentally. The first chakra is the red chakra, or the root chakra. This is the root chakra because it is the one that is responsible for helping you become aware of yourself and your mental state.

You will need to determine the ways that you will open the chakra as well. This guide has presented you with the many different ways that this can be done. It is important that you focus on each of them and ensure that you are prepared. You must be willing to do them all in order to attain the best amount of success possible. As we have mentioned time and time again, yoga is one of the very best ways that you can become in tune with the seven chakras that are found within your body.

It is usually with the help of your instructor that you learn the best ways of becoming in tune with your chakras. For most people it takes years and years of practice in order to be able to gain a full sense of wellbeing with the chakras. Once you have gained the proper instruction and have begun to feel energized through the different chakras it is then that you may be able to start doing things on your own.

Learning your chakras, as well as how to become in tune with them, is certainly a life changing experience. It can change your entire persona, the whole person that you are. It isn't for those who aren't truly focused upon becoming a success however; so make sure that you are committed from the start.

As you learn the different chakras and yoga techniques to perform them you will be able to become a new you, the person that you always wanted to be, the person that you knew was there but did not know how to break out. It is something that can now be done if you can connect to yourself: body, mind and soul.

Benefits of Chakra Yoga

As one might expect, there are a number of benefits that come along with the introduction of yoga to enhance the various chakras within the body. All of these exciting benefits come to those who are regular participants in the form of yoga. It is not difficult at all to start participating in this form of yoga. And anyone who is feeling down, like they are not themselves, should participate in the form of yoga to benefit him or herself.

The benefits of yoga on the chakras in the body may come slowly, and that is okay. It takes time, effort and diligence in order to overcome some of the various aspects of our lives.

How do you know that your chakras are out of whack and in need of a bit of adjustment? It is usually not very difficult to determine that something isn't right. People who have imbalances of the chakra are depressed, sad, angry and otherwise do not feel good about themselves. You may not have the energy to do things during the day that you would normally love to participate in. You might find yourself no longer enjoying these activities and instead choosing to avoid them. Another symptom that is indicative of chakras that are not well balanced: you might find yourself lashing out at the people that you love the most, or feeling a mound of health problems on a regular basis. If you are not full of life, full of energy and mentally sound, one or more of the chakras may be out of line and may need improvement.

With the regular use of chakra an individual can heal him or herself and feel better than ever before. In the previous chapter, we discussed some of the pitfalls that come along with the chakras when they are imbalanced, and laid it all out on the line to heal you. All of this can be done without the use of medications that can cause the body harm, and it brings a heightened sense of self-awareness. All of the benefits that have already been listed in thief guide are the things that you can experience when you begin to intertwine with your mind and your body through this alternate yoga technique.

Through the regular use of yoga, all of these chakras can become balanced and you can build yourself spiritually. Yoga enables you to feel good about yourself, mentally and physically. It eliminates many health problems that so many people face, and it also enables you to become more aware of your being.

If you have any of the problems that we have listed already in this guide, there is a good chance that your chakras are imbalanced. Rather than go from doctor to doctor to doctor getting various diagnoses and medications (which, if you did not already know, can cause an abundance of problems within themselves) you can be participating in yoga and eliminate those worries while healing yourself.

Let's examine some more of the exciting benefits of chakra yoga.

Improved Blood Circulation: Through the performance of yoga you are improving the blood circulation. When this happens you can help minimize infections as well as the amount of toxins that are flowing through your body.

You will feel good participating in chakra yoga. All of the senses of the body are found within these regions of the body. When they are in balance, you feel good, you feel energetic and ready to take on the world.

When the chakras are well balanced you are able to feel good about yourself, and you are a more caring and considerate person to other people.

People who participate in this kind of yoga are able to eliminate many of the aches and pains that they feel. Many of these types of complaints are really there, but they are enhanced by the mind and the mental thought and process. Once it is balanced, as it should be, the yoga is able to provide astonishing benefits that influence everyone greatly.

It is possible to lose weight when participating in this form of yoga. Although most doctors or personal trainers do not recommend yoga as a method of weight loss, there are some types of yoga, those known as high intensity yoga, that can work greatly to help shed the weight right off.

Are you stressed out? Do you need a way to relax and unwind? This is yet another exciting benefit that comes along with the practice of yoga to open the chakras of the body.

Yoga enables your body to do great things, and it is only with the power of the mind that these things are possible to happen. You will feel more energized and can move around better when you are performing yoga. If you have back pains and aches, headaches or migraines or otherwise feel that you are 'stiff,' participating in yoga can turn your life around.

This is just a partial list of the many ways that you can benefit yourself with the use of yoga to energize and enhance the chakras. It is in your best interest to learn more about chakra and begin initiating it into your life as quickly as you possibly can.

When you use yoga to develop your chakras you can improve relationships with all individuals in your life. This includes your parents, children, co-workers and of course your spouse. With the development of the senses of the chakra you can learn how to feel less needy and become a more supportive person for those around you as well as be able to put things into a better prospective when there is conflict occurring. You will learn how to attract people that you want to be in your life and will even be able to find sexual relationships more gratifying for yourself. Finally, you can learn how to become a good listener, a quality that we all probably could stand a bit of working on.

When you are in tune with all of your senses, those seven found within the chakra, you are able to understand other people as well as the energy that they have within them. You understand that you are energy as is the next person, and learn how to complement the energy of other people rather than take it back. You can learn how to properly mix energies so that you can connect, and always take a breath of fresh air at the end of the day.

Since you are healing on all levels with energizing the chakras, you are able to stop suffering that hurt. You can do this, according to the philosophies of yoga, when you transcend yourself and your mind into the cycle of samsara.

So, to sum it up, the following benefits of chakra improvement are found:

- ✓ *Help eliminate hurt and pain*
- ✓ *Strength to carry on to another day*
- ✓ *Depression, anxiety treatment*
- ✓ *Better appetite*
- ✓ *Better digestion*
- ✓ *Improvement in relationships*
- ✓ *Better overall health*
- ✓ *More energy*
- ✓ *More positivity*
- ✓ *Add creativity and spark to your imagination*

These are just some of the exciting benefits that come along with chakra energizing and yoga. Make sure that you are participating in it on a regular basis and enjoying each and every one of these benefits for yourself. They are there and they are waiting for you if you are willing to take advantage of them. What are you waiting for? What is there to lose?

Enhancing the Chakras with Yoga

When any of these seven different chakras are not in tune as they should be, many problems can and will occur. They affect each person in a different manner, but it is safe to say that none of them are very desirable. When your chakras are not in tune it can cause a big disruption to your life, the relationships that you have with other people and more.

Being in tune with the chakras is not something that everyone can do, but it is certainly a possibility that they have. It is up to that person, however, to understand the chakras and how they affect them. Once this information is understood the person is able to energize the chakras within them and start making the changes that are necessary to revive and energize themselves into better people all the way around.

While an individual can choose to do this in any number of different ways, it is with the assistance of yoga that the ultimate results can be found. Yoga is definitely a technique that you must work to learn, but in the end it is very much wroth the troubles. You will look better, feel better and have a better mentality all the way around.

Mediation is an important part of yoga, but there are many different attributes that each of them bring forth. Yoga enables the individual to feel better physically and emotionally, where mediation focuses only on the mental state of an individual.

It is always best to seek the help of a certified yoga instructor to help you get started with yoga. The yoga instructor is already well aware of their chakras and how to entice them through the help of yoga. They can spread their expertise on to you so that you are able to become aware of the senses and what they mean to you.

Once the proper yoga training and instruction has been provided, you can then take your needs to your own home or other place of choice and participate on your own and with your own time. It is at that point that you will be aware of your senses, each of the 7 chakras, as well as how to fine-tune your inner being to them.

Your physical energy is your aura. It is the psychic energy produced by life force, and it is around you in all forms, including physical, mentally and emotionally. There are several different colors associated with the aura, which represent your mood. It is important, however, to understand that the auras are constantly changing and can strengthen or change size at any time. Your aura affects your wellbeing and your mental state.

Finding The Right Yoga Instructor

Hatha is the most commonly chosen type of yoga performed by beginners and individuals who are ready to tune into their energy and chakras. It enlists the basic yoga moves and helps familiarize the individual with the techniques and the various moves. We all know that yoga can take time to master, thus starting off with this form is an excellent idea. Of course, if you prefer to do something else it is completely up to you, but it is important that you are aware of the types that are out there, and the one that you want to do. Not all yoga instructors or studios offer the same type of instruction, thus making sure of what you want and what you are getting ahead of time is a must.

There are many ways to research the various types of yoga out there, as well as their benefits and how they can help you regain the lost energy with the chakras. This includes using the Internet, researching history journals and publications and of course through research papers. Yoga has a very interesting history, and dates back for centuries in Chinese medicine. It is very interesting to learn and it can help you out as you advance.

Make sure that you take the time to visit the website of any instructor that you are considering. On the website you can learn a wide variety of information about the center, including the year that it started and the different types of yoga that they are offering to the world. You might also want to use the web to find reviews of the center from people who have firsthand experience using the company. There are various websites that offer testimonials and other information about the yoga instruction, and with this information you can benefit yourself greatly.

Next, research the various yoga studios near your. Most people choose a center that is close in proximity to work or school since this makes thing sore convenient. However, you are always free to choose where you will go for yoga. While you are searching for studios in your area, make sure that you are also getting to know more about them through the same resources as mentioned above. You do not want to trust your alternative health means to just anyone, and with so many different resource to help you, there is no reason to do so.

What should you seek to find when choosing your yoga studio? It is far more than the convenient location (which, of course, we hope that you are able to find.)

You must also take the time to learn yoga etiquette. It is very important to familiar yourself with this so you won't feel so out of place while in class and also to give yourself an advantage to some of the others. The etiquette of yoga must be followed with each class. It is all a part of freeing yourself; body, mind and soul.

The cost of the class is another concern that many people have, and yet another reason that comparing is so important to do. Not all classes will cost the same amount of money; so if you are worried about this at all, make sure that you are aware of the prices ahead of time. Most studios have their prices listed on their website if you take a look. If you are not on the web or prefer to speak to someone in person, this is also possible and they will be more than happy to inform you of the prices that you will pay for the specifics that you are interested in.

It is very important that you take your classes and the instruction very seriously. Yoga is not for the weak hearted and must be followed precisely for the full benefits to result. It is for those who truly want to change their mind and become in tune with their inner being.

What is an Aura?

Everything in the universe is just a vibration. Every atom, part of an atom, electron, proton, and neutron is a vibration of energy. Even your thoughts are a vibration of energy. Light and sound are simple examples of a vibration of energy. If you took a metal rod and began to shake it, as it speeds up, it will produce sound. If you were able to speed it up even more, eventually it will produce heat and light.

An Aura is an electro-photonic vibration response of an object to some external excitation. An aura surrounds every living thing in the universe. Human aura has layers of emotional, mental, physical, and spiritual elements. The aura around conscious or living beings may very with time. They can also change very quickly and rapidly. The aura around non-living beings remains fixed and may be altered by conscious intent.

Auras are made up of all the primary colors of the rainbow at any given time and may change their color depending upon the emotions that are being experienced. Your aura is therefore made up of various shades of colors that change constantly. This change demonstrates the constant alterations in your emotions and thoughts.

The most important thing about an aura is the fact that in contains every bit of information about an object. The intensity and the color of the aura, especially above and surrounding your head has a definite meaning. Learning the skills of watching someone's aura can enable you to experience someone thoughts before they express them verbally. It is very easy to spot liars because an aura can't be faked.

Your aura is your spiritual signature.

Let's examine the different auras and colors associated with them.

Blue: If you have a blue aura, you are balanced, without stress and at ease in all faucets in your life. Everyone wants to have the blue aura. For those who are clairvoyant, the blue aura can also come their way when communication with the dead is taking place.

Purple: if the aura is purple there is an indication of a spiritual being within in. Sometimes purple appears in flashes or in flames only.

Green: another color of aura is green. This color is also desirable and indicated natural energy that is needed for healing. Those who have a green aura are rested, healed on the inside and are oftentimes those who are good at gardening, or have a green thumb.

Turquoise: those with this color aura are dynamic individuals who are energetic and great thinkers. It is those with the turquoise aura that are usually influencing the decisions of other people. Turquoise aura indicated that a person is organized and has goals in place.

Yellow is a bright color that means you are joyful and spiritual. People who have this color aura are generous human beings.

Orange: Orange is another aura color that you might have. If you do, it is a sign that you are a powerful individual and you would not have things any other way. It is something that you enjoy and desire to have such power.

Red: The final aura color is red. If you have an aura that is red you are a materialistic person who dwells upon him or herself. You are someone that thinks highly of himself or herself and cares about his or her appearance greatly.

Final Words: Thank you!

 I hope this book was able to help you to learn more about what the chakras are and how they affect your overall wellbeing. We also hope that you were able to find great tips to help you transform your life and turn things around. Anyone has the power to make this connection if they are willing to make it. One of the best ways that this can be done is through the practice of yoga. There are millions of people who participate in yoga around the world. Take a look at any of them and you will notice they certainly have a great energy, vibe or an aura about them. You want to be the same type of persona and it is possible if you get in touch with your chakra.

The next step is to take things into your own hands and learn more about chakras and how they can help you through the use of yoga. There are so many exciting benefits that come with yoga, and it is when you begin performing these various exercises that you can turn your whole life around. When you are able to energize the chakras and participate in yoga at the same time you are certainly getting the best of both worlds and will feel better than what you ever have before.

Finally, if you enjoyed this book, please take the time to share your thoughts and post a review on Amazon. It'd be greatly appreciated!

ABAHA SAAGAR

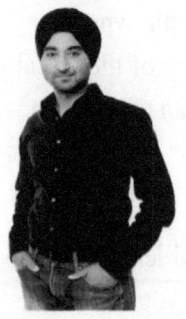

About The Author: Abaha was born in Karnataka India. He is a graduate of the Binar School of Yoga in India. For graduate school, Abaha moved to America to attend the Hindu University of America in Orlando, Florida. He did not plan on staying in America after graduation, but fell in love with the American culture. He recognized an opportunity to teach, and currently provides classes on a wide range of topics. His focus is Kundalini Yoga, and his philosophy of topics include the chakra energy systems; studies in raja, bhakti, jnana, and karma yoga; Ayurveda; Hindu spirituality; Buddhism spirituality and classes in Sanskrit, and the Vedas.

"Your environment is a force that attempts to break the link between your mind and body, but Yoga mends the mind and body together in harmony."

Here are some other great reads from Abaha Saagar:

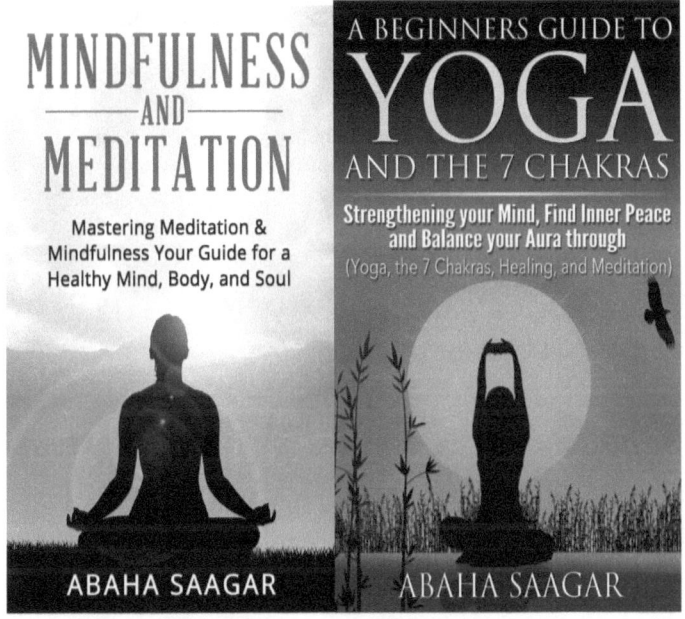

Copyright © 2014

Disclaimer

www.ingramcontent.com/pod-product-compliance
Lightning Source LLC
Chambersburg PA
CBHW030542290526
45786CB00004B/1819